Lecture Reprint Number 4

A NEW SLANT ON HEALTH AND BEAUTY (Slant Board)

by Bernard Jensen, Ph.D., D.C., N.D.

Revised and edited by Jon D. Jensen

ACKNOWLEDGEMENTS

I acknowledge and give thanks to Betty Norlin for being such a wonderful friend and for continually encouraging me and assisting me on my book writing/editing journey. Author of *"Our Bodies: The Optimal Design."*

www.bettynorlin.com   www.whatisholistichealth.com

I acknowledge and give thanks to Daylin Anderson for editing and compiling information for this lecture reprint booklet series.

I acknowledge and give thanks to Gary and Jeanne Nichols. They have given their expertise in editing and marketing as well as assisting me with my grandfather's videos taking them from video to DVD. They have always supported me whether it was creating an office space, writing, or giving lectures. Thank you both!

COPYRIGHT

Copyright @ 2021 by Jon D. Jensen

Because of the dynamic nature of the Internet, any web addresses or links contained in this book may have changed since publication and may no longer be valid.

Paperback

ISBN-9781688464360

4

DISCLAIMER

Any information given in this book is not intended to be taken as a replacement for medical advice. Any person with a condition requiring medical attention should consult a qualified health professional.

INTRODUCTION

My name is Jon Jensen and I have been involved in the holistic health field for many years. I published a nutrition book, *"A Simple Guide to Healthy Living"* as a way to communicate with people outside my client base about information I feel is key to a healthy life. It is available on Amazon or through my website, www.jensenholistichealth.com.

I've had the idea to publish these health booklets for many years. My intention for editing, revising and publishing my grandfather's 21 lecture reprint booklets is rooted in my desire to continue his legacy of teaching right living through health and nutrition. Dr. Bernard Jensen spent his lifetime helping others to achieve health through education and his writing, and I feel strongly that the message is needed now more than ever.

I've always marveled how one person could write so many books and still travel, receive numerous awards, teach classes on Iridology, rejuvenation, regeneration and tissue cleansing. He recorded his lectures onto cassette tapes and eventually had a series of videos that corresponded to many of his books. These lecture reprints are the product of his first lectures, typed up and stapled into booklets and originally sold for ninety-nine cents each. Thus started a pattern where he would write and self-publish many books over his lifetime. He did end up publishing books with a couple publishing companies, but most of his work was self-published.

Bernard Jensen, Ph.D., D.C., N.D.

One of the greatest healers the world has ever known. Dr. Bernard Jensen spent over 60 years as a pioneer in the holistic health field, helping to pave the way for the alternative health revolution that we are now experiencing.

Dr. Jensen began his career at the West Coast Chiropractic College where he became the youngest Chiropractor in the state of California. He traveled extensively in search of health knowledge, a search that led him to over 65 countries to observe the lifestyles of the people and their various ways of eating. Each place provided a different health secret.

Throughout his career, Dr. Jensen wrote and published over 60 books, a quarterly magazine for several years, a cassette and video tape series and a slide presentation for his Iridology class. After working with over 350,000 patients, Dr. Jensen firmly believed that nutrition is the greatest single therapy to be applied in the holistic healing arts and that, "We must treat the patient, not just the disease."

Born on March 25, 1908, to parents of Danish descent, Eugen and Anna Jensen, Jorgen Bernard Jensen was raised in Stockton, California, then a small rural town in one of the richest agricultural valleys of the state. The unexpected death of his mother at age 29 from tuberculosis and consumption left the three children to be raised by their father, Eugen Jensen who was a chiropractor. Very little has been written about Bernard's early life growing up in Stockton, his brother and sister, and a few comments in lectures he made about his father who was mentioned as very strict and analytical.

Early in life, young Bernard displayed the qualities needed for his future work. His penchant for being an analytical, critical, serious perfectionist blended with his sensitive, competitive, spiritual-minded personality to arm him with an unusual perspective that opened the doors to the unconventional life he was soon to enter. But before that path was firmly set, several intense learning experiences occurred which determined the direction he was to take.

Being his own worst obstacle, restless and never satisfied, he would rather study and read a book than eat or sleep. His father was a chiropractor, and young Bernard followed in his path. When he was 18 years old, Bernard entered the West Coast Chiropractic College in Oakland, California. During his years of study, Bernard burned the midnight oil while holding down as many as two outside jobs simultaneously. The strain was immense. The capacity to push forward and the ability to persevere doggedly toward a goal were firmly established, but there was a price to pay. Bernard supported himself by working at a dairy in his spare time, and the long hours of work and study, along with poor food habits, took a heavy toll on Bernard's health. After receiving his diploma in 1929, Dr. Bernard Jensen went into practice, opening his first office in Oakland, California. He focused intently on the task of his calling which was to offer a helping hand to those suffering and in need. Dr. Bernard Jensen's devotion was complete, the hours long, his personal needs forgotten. By this time, the sacrificing of many years began to demand attention. His health began to fail. A Medical Doctor diagnosed his condition as bronchiectasis, an often-fatal lung condition, with no known cure at the time. "There is nothing I can do for you," he was told.

The young man refused to give up, searching out a Seventh Day Adventist Medical Doctor who taught him basic nutritional principles, told Dr. Bernard Jensen to leave junk food alone and promptly presented him with a maintenance program involving natural health that emphasized the return to a pure, natural and whole foods regimen. Following this program brought excellent results. Dr. Bernard Jensen was soon on the way back to health and renewed vitality. A great turning point had occurred. To be able to study nutrition and discover the laws of right living became his burning desire. Dr. Bernard Jensen turned the experience of what he learned from the Seventh Day Adventist Medical Doctor about the holistic approach into helping his patients get better and teach them how to prevent themselves from getting sick. Dr. Bernard Jensen began taking breathing exercises with Thomas Gaines, once an instructor for the New York City Police Department. Slowly, his health returned, and his lungs eventually healed completely.

Using this knowledge in working with his patients the results were dramatic and effective. Dr. Bernard Jensen's attention was now riveted in this direction. Natural therapeutics became his healing mode, setting the pattern for the rest of his life. He began to travel in search of more knowledge and information.

Dr. Bernard Jensen opened his first office in Oakland, California, in 1929. He later moved to Los Angeles and expanded his practice to include branch offices at Long Beach and Santa Monica, with several chiropractors working under him. Such success had not come about overnight. In Chicago, Dr. Bernard Jensen took his post-graduate work at the National Chiropractic College and later from the Los Angeles Chiropractic College closer to home. Upon returning to California, he began an intensive study and investigation of something he was recently just learning about, the subject of iridology.

Dr. Bernard Jensen used Rocine's work as the basis for the programs used in his sanitariums. First, a 25-bed sanitarium in San Leandro, California, then others in Ben Lomond and Alta Dena, and finally an 85-bed sanitarium at hidden Valley Health Ranch in Escondido, California. The sanitariums were quite successful, demonstrating the effectiveness of Rocine's ideas in working with patients. It was the Hidden Valley Health Ranch in Escondido that provided the greatest opportunity for applying the rules of right living. People in search of health and rejuvenation came to the ranch from all over the world to learn the principles that Dr. Bernard Jensen believed in, practiced, and taught.

Proper nutrition, together with sunshine, rest, exercise, fresh air and positive attitudes helped thousands of patients at Dr. Bernard Jensen's sanitariums leave behind the symptoms of chronic diseases that they have developed. After working with several hundred thousand patients, Dr. Bernard Jensen concluded that nutrition is the single most important therapy to be used in the healing arts.

Patients came from all over the world, some to stay at his sanitariums, others for outpatient consultations and still others to attend his classes in rejuvenation and Food Studies. Thousands of New Zealanders formed clubs to follow his dietetic advice, filling out the over 350,000 people he reached, accumulated over the years. He acquired a multitude of experiences from these people individually and in group studies, acquiring information and summing it up for use in his healing work and writing.

Dr. Bernard Jensen visited the Hunza Valley, where disease, doctors, dentist and hospitals were practically nonexistent and where there were no jails, prisons or police, because there was no crime. One of Dr. Bernard Jensen's highlights of that trip was staying as a guest of the Mir of Hunza's palace for 10 days.

Dr. Bernard Jensen visited the Caucasus Mountains in the USSR to meet a 153-year-old man who had stopped riding horseback a few years earlier only because of his doctor's orders. Dr. Bernard Jensen traveled to Vilcabamba, Ecuador, where heart patients were able to recuperate so marvelously. Everywhere Dr. Bernard Jensen went, he brought back some new remedy or approach to integrate into the system he taught his patients.

Dr. Bernard Jensen received his Ph.D. at the age of 75 from the University of Humanistic Studies, San Diego, California.

Dr. Bernard Jensen retired from active chiropractic practice in 1978, and devoted himself to teaching, writing and lecturing on the subjects of nutrition, rejuvenation and iridology. Around this time, Dr. Bernard Jensen completed work on a two-hour feature film titled, *"World Search for Health, Happiness and Long Life,"* narrated by actor Dennis Weaver.

The Academy of Science in Paris awarded Dr. Bernard Jensen a medal in 1971 for exceptional services rendered to humanity. Also, in the same year, 1971, Dr. Bernard Jensen received an honorary doctorate from the Center for the Study of Human Sciences in Lisbon, Portugal.

At a ceremony in San Remo, Italy in 1973, Dr. Bernard Jensen was presented the Ignatz Von Peczely International Iridology Gold Medal by the World Congress of Scientific Medicine, an organization embracing many medical and health disciplines.

A congress of health professionals at Aix-en Provence, France, in 1974, recognized Dr. Bernard Jensen with an award for his "valuable contribution in the field of iridology."

Then in 1975, the International Naturopathic Association honored Dr. Bernard Jensen for his service to mankind through his work in the fields of health,

Iridology, and nutrition.

Knighted into the Order of St. John of Malta in 1978 for his humanitarian work in the field of health, Dr. Bernard Jensen was awarded the cross of St. John at a special ceremony in New York City. This Order is the oldest chivalric organization in the world, tracing its origin back to the time preceding the first Crusade.

In 1981, at the Fifth Annual Herb Symposium, the Agnes Arber Distinguished Service award was presented to Dr. Bernard Jensen for his contributions to the current "herb renaissance."

In 1982, the National Health Federation honored Dr. Bernard Jensen with its Pioneer Doctor of the Year award at its annual convention in Long Beach, California.

In 1982, Dr. Bernard Jensen traveled to Brussels, Belgium to accept the 1982 Dag Hammarskjold award of the Pax Mundi Academy, an international organization which presents annual awards to those in the arts and sciences who have made outstanding contributions in their fields. The award, in the category of scientific merit, was for "the exceptional services rendered to collective humanity... toward international cooperation and solidarity..." Dr. Bernard Jensen was personally congratulated on his award by U. S. Ambassador, Charles Price.

In 1988 Dr. Bernard Jensen held his 80th Birthday Celebration at the Town and Country Hotel in San Diego, California, where people came from all over the world to celebrate his 80 years of life and work in the holistic health field.

In 1993 he was presented with a PhD. in natural healing arts and sciences from Westbrook University, where his iridology course was part of the school curriculum.

In 1995 Dr. Bernard Jensen's grandson Jon stayed by his grandfather's side after Dr. Jensen became paralyzed from the waist down from a car accident. Jon was right there every day of his grandfather's plan to walk again. With a big sign on the wall in front of Dr. Jensen's bed where he could see it every day that said, "LUCKY BOY." Every day consisted of many different healing modalities and supplements. Jon would travel to the Hidden Valley Health Ranch in the early morning and watch while Apolinar, Dr. Jensen's main ranch worker, milked the goat for Dr. Jensen's fresh morning goat milk drink. After breakfast and supplements, there was stretching, going to the gym and massages 2 times a week. A physical therapist came in every day to assist in the gym and to stretch the muscles. Jon would drive his grandfather and grandmother Marie to Los Angeles twice a week for chiropractic adjustments and frequency therapy, treating the whole body, mind, and spirit, and being involved in every aspect of what the doctors called a **"Miracle"—as his grandfather walked again on his own.** Jon is writing more on the entire recovery process and will publish it through Amazon.

In 1998 and 1999 Dr. Bernard Jensen received awards from the IIPA for his work in iridology.

On February 22, 2001 a month before his 93rd birthday, Dr. Bernard Jensen passed away at 92 years old.

The short biography above about Dr. Bernard Jensen is a small part of a larger biography I am writing about my grandfather's life. If you are interested in learning more I will be blogging and have more information at www.bernardjensen.org.

In the 21 lecture reprint booklets you'll see products or foods that might not be commonly found today. I left some things in to give the flavor of that time period and what he was thinking at that time. I also left in quotes or sayings from that era. I edited misspellings and grammatical errors. But overall, I feel that these booklets give down to earth advice and can still be regarded as basic knowledge in the mainstream health field today. A lot of his products are no longer available, but you can find what remains on my website, www.jensenholistichealth.com.

I hope you enjoy these lecture reprint booklets as much as I do and take them for what they are. If nothing else, a novelty and glimpse of the past. A simple approach of one of the early promoters of healthy living. Alongside such greats of that era like Paul Bragg, Jack LaLanne, Dr. Max Gerson, V.E. Irons and Dr. Bronner at the beginning of a health revolution.

Jon D. Jensen, CMH

A NEW SLANT ON HEALTH AND BEAUTY (Slant Board)

"My purpose is to serve and I must serve my purpose."

Bernard Jensen, Ph.D., D.C., N.D.

There are natural laws of nature by which we all live and which we all live, and which greatly affect our daily lives. The sun rises in the morning, travels its course of the day and sets in the evening. It is an inevitable cycle. The moon rises and sets and the tides are affected by the moon's cycle. There are some tides that rise to a height of sixteen feet. Gravity pulls this tide of water down again when the pull of the moon is taken away. The same effect is produced on our body. The universe produces cycles of gravity in our body. These things are unchangeable; they will always be, and so, when we recognize the effect they have on our lives, we can adjust ourselves to them.

Gravity is a law of nature that affects the human body just as much as it affects the trees and plant life. We cannot escape from this inevitable law of nature, and so we should adapt ourselves to some procedure whereby we can overcome any ill effects we might suffer because of the effects of this law. The pull of gravity is always downward; the river flows downstream; the bird, when he loses his energy, drops back to the earth; the blade of grass, when not properly nourished, turns back into the earth. Man exists under this law also and, if he is tired and exhausted, he feels the pull of gravity pulling him down he wishes to lie down and rest. When a person is full of pep and energy he stands upright, walks with zest, has a good posture and develops tone in every muscle of his body which holds all of the organs in the proper position. He is the master, as he is meant to be; he has control of his body; he is greater than the law of gravity.

The man who has lost his energy through improper diet, over-indulgence and through a lack of mental ease in his life, finally falls prey to the law of gravity. He is unable to carry on his work or to live as he should. In order to make a success of life, we must know these universal laws and conform to them. Let us learn to recognize these natural laws and set ourselves up to live by them and also to overcome any ill effects that may have resulted from disobeying these laws.

If people would only live happily, they would remain well. There is an old Hebrew saying: "A merry heart causeth good healing, but a broken spirit drieth up the bones." How true this is. If we learn to live constructively, with good food, exercise and proper breathing, nothing would ever go wrong with our body. The body is the most amazing machine that has ever been constructed and the work that it does in repairing itself is almost unbelievable. God, who created this wonderful mechanism, is also able to maintain it in perfection, if we follow His natural laws.

Our modern civilization creates a driving force in our bodies. We are anxious about almost everything.

Desires, with anxiety, produce acids in the body. Anger creates sickness; jealousy and hatred break down the body. Fighting the day is only fighting one's self. We must learn to discipline ourselves, for to master one's self is to master all of gravity. There is not a single disease you can name in which gravity does not play a part. We must recognize that this law exists, and we cannot change it. You will never be able to change the pull on your body, because this law is fixed. It is so much a part of the universe that you must learn to live with it.

There is only one thing you can do with this law of gravity and that is to work with it. You will have to change yourself. First, by lying down, as there is less pull on the flow of blood in your body that there would be if you were standing up or sitting down. The pull is only eight inches, while if you are standing up, it can be a five or six foot pull on the flow of blood in the body. While you are lying down, gravity is pulling the blood to the upper part of your body, which will get a good deal of blood to the cerebellum, or back part of the brain. You need to regenerate the physical part of your body, so it is necessary to lie down and get the head below the rest of the body so that gravity will pull the blood down to the back and the lower part of the head. The cerebellum is the physical part of the brain center where every physical organ of your body is regenerated. You could not move your toe without this back part of your brain working properly. You could not move your fingers if the back brain did not have all the blood it needed to carry the necessary nerve force. You could not breathe without the proper quantity of blood in the back part of the brain. The brain and the head are the uppermost parts of the body and when gravity pulls on us when we are walking around, the first part of the body to be affected is the brain area and the head.

Several years ago, I came across some ideas on gravity which I will give you to show the value of this. I know that what I tell you will prove itself. The reason I know this is because I have been my own guinea pig. I was not endowed with such a perfect body that I could say "Look at me." I have had to work for my health, and I must continue to do the right thing in order to keep my health. In the year 1933 I was very ill. I had considerable rectal and lower bowel troubles of a very serious nature. I had to go through a crisis. I lived thirteen days on grapes and a day came when, during the crisis, I had to overcome this problem by getting in an upside-down position. At that moment I recognized that I had found something. It was not new; other people had talked of it before, but I do not think anyone experienced it more clearly than I. I do not think anyone needed it more than I did the night I went through the crisis. This great need of mine, during this illness, showed me the value in the use of the slanting board. I found, through necessity, one of the greatest means of correcting our health problems and help in maintaining a healthy body.

The use of the slanting board, from that time on, has become a daily habit with me and is one of the means of relaxation and exercise that I give all my patients as a regular part of their "get well and stay well" program.

The slanting board need not be an elaborate affair. We have some beautiful models with plush coverings, some that are the folding type, but these are the luxury kind, nice to have, but not necessary. The use of some kind of a board is necessary for health, however. You can even use your ironing board, or any kind of a board on which you can lie with your feet higher than your head. The back of a chair will suffice, if you have no board.

A slanting board should be from eighteen to twenty inches wide, six feet long and made of five-ply wood, three-fourths of an inch thick. Side handles may be made by cutting holes in the board three-quarters of an inch in from the edge, or by adding handles that are nailed to the underside of the board about midway down on the board. Straps should be fastened near the foot of the board to hold the ankles in place for the exercises, so that the body will not slide down and so that you can pull up to a sitting position. A prop under the board should be set so that the foot end will be about eighteen inches higher than the head. If this prop is not added on to the board itself, the board may be propped up to these eighteen inches higher than the head. If this prop is not added on to the board itself, the board may be propped up to this eighteen-inch height by allowing the foot end of the board to rest on some object that height from the floor.

The daily use of a slanting board will help any condition that is wrong in the body. It allows all organs to be moved back into their proper positions, particularly the prolapsed organs, and starts the flow of blood into the head and brain area. It is impossible to overemphasize the importance of getting blood into all the extremities. The brain is the center of our living; all movements emanate from the brain first and if it is blood starved, we naturally have slow reactions in other parts of the body.

I know that unless there is proper blood in the head, you cannot have proper eyesight; your ears cannot have proper hearing; you cannot taste properly; you cannot think properly. The average person who has an anemic condition of the brain because of lack of blood flowing to the brain, caused by gravity, always has a poor memory and an inability to make decisions. He is not as quick as he formerly was. When these symptoms appear, he needs a slanting board. I have never yet found a person who did not have some prolapsus; therefore, I have never found a person who did not need a slanting board. Every patient of mine uses a board, or he is not my patient. If a person does as I tell him, he improves. I can only tell you the right things to do, then you must do them yourself. No one can get you well but yourself. There is no nurse who will do as much for you as you can yourself, if you have the knowledge.

I have had many boards made by Mr. Pierce who regained his health by the use of the board. He was in his seventies when he first saw me demonstrating the board at the Hollywood Roosevelt Hotel. He has carried the message of what the board will do too many thousands of people. He is past eighty and attributes his vibrant health, to the use of the slanting board.

Everyone should lie on the slanting board every afternoon. About three o'clock there is a change in the moon and sun and when we have that change, the fluids and the pull in the body are making a change also. If we did not have to carry on at that time and were able to take care of that pull by allowing gravity to do its constructive work while in an upside-down position, we would find we would not have much trouble the rest of the day.

When I come home from work and get on the slanting board before dinner, even for five minutes, I can go to the table and be so relaxed that my food is a great deal more satisfactory to me. The greatest sin we can possibly commit against the body is to go to bed with prolapsed organs and wake up the next day with organs in the same position. Doing this, day after day, causes adhesions and trouble in the abdominal tract. When you get into bed, lift the buttocks, pull the organs into their proper position and lie down. You recuperate most when you are sleeping so allow these tissues to recuperate in their natural position. Why allow them to relax in a prolapsed position? It is a wonderful feeling to know that you are starting the day with all organs in their natural position. No matter what your condition is, the slanting board will definitely help it.

The slanting board will do many things for you. One of my patients came to me with eye trouble. I have a letter in my office from a Dr. Jacques, an optometrist in Los Angeles, who wrote that He could not understand why he had to change the glasses of a lady after a period of only four months' time. I advised him that the change was due to the eye exercises she did, but I give the slanting board the greatest credit because the eye exercises were more effective, having been practiced while she reclined on the slanting board.

Another patient whose sight was improved through the use of the slanting board is the twelve-year-old son of Mr. and Mrs. Block who own the health food store on LA Brea and Wilshire, Los Angeles. In four months, he raised his vision from forty percent to one hundred percent. He removed his glasses entirely. The slanting board was responsible for most of that.

We have colored moving pictures of a lady who had grey hair when she came to us and in one month's time her hair turned completely yellow through a Sulphur elimination which was working out through the hair during the elimination process: However, in another month's time that grey hair turned to black again. The hair was stimulated through a flow of blood to the scalp through the persistent use of the slanting board.

Joe Tonti, the strong upside-down man featured by Ripley in "Believe It or Not," had many abnormal symptoms involving ears, eyes and head. He also lost his hair but regained it after spending most of his time exercising and working in an upside-down position.

The slanting board is not something to be used only for a specific condition of the body. It is good for the eyes, ears, nose, toenails, hair, or anything you can mention. When I take care of the body, I do not treat just the bowel or the eyes. I treat the whole body and the slant board is one of my best friends for treating the body. A cure comes when new tissue takes the place of the old tissue. When you are trying to get well, learn everything that is needed and do all the things required and you will get well.

Most of the symptoms of disease are started in a tired body. Weger, in his "Control and Genesis of Disease," say's to consider when we are trying to get our bodies well. When we are tired, do we rest? We are all taught that achievement and accomplishment must be undertaken. If we say we will be somewhere at eight o'clock and come home half-dead at 7:30, we still drag ourselves there. How many people have a job where they can quit at two or three o'clock because they feel tired? The pressure of everyday life does not allow us to do these things.

One point I would like to bring out here is: that in my study of Iridiagnosis, I found that the chart indicates that the upper part of the eye represents the brain area. In the very center of the brain area of the eye is the fatigue center, straight up at the twelve o'clock point. This represents the topmost part of the brain. Whenever we have a condition of old age setting in, there is a ring in the eye called the Arcus Senilis, Arc of Senility, or the Arc of Old Age. This arc of Old Age is the same as any anemic condition, only it is in the brain and not in the rest of the body. This Arc of Senilis has its greatest width in the topmost part of the eye, which has its greatest effect in the fatigue center. The fatigue center is the first thing affected when the Arc of Senilis has its beginning. Fatigue is the first thing we should correct in getting well. Rest cures; doctors do not.

This fatigue center is the greatest barometer in the body. You should follow it. Your body knows best what you should do for it. Many times I think it would have been to our benefit if we were constructed in such a way that we could knock ourselves out so that we would have to lie down when we were tired, because a strong will power will just keep us going on, for the simple reason that we were taught to "keep going." Very few people have been taught to stop, relax and let-go, schools do not teach these things. We seldom give the body a change to recuperate when it desires to go through its recuperative period. Fatigue is the one thing that sins against man more than anything else because fatigue produces no pain in the body and so we fight it and work against it. There is always so much to do and to see that we do not stop when we are tired.

A tired heart cannot pump blood very hard. Arteries were made to contract, but tired tissues in the arteries cannot contract enough to force the blood against gravity uphill to the brain area. Therefore, we have anemic tissues in the brain areas. Since we do everything from the brain, move our fingers, move our feet, etc., they all depend upon the blood that is in the head and upon the amount of recuperation that has set in during the night and day. If gravity is the force that keeps pulling down when we are standing up, thus causing the trouble, why not get the head down and work along with this gravity pull?

We now have the correction and the correction is found in going along with this natural law of gravity. If it has pulled on you while you were standing on your feet, and pulled everything down towards the lower extremities, this same law can be utilized by turning yourself upside down and allowing the law of gravity to pull the other way, putting all the organs back into their normal position, and pulling the blood into the brain which was made anemic in the upright position. The foregoing should show you the importance of the use of the slanting board in the "get well" program. I now want to give some specific diseases and suggested exercises that will help in overcoming these diseases.

BLOOD PRESSURE

Blood pressure should run 120, no matter what the age. When the blood vessels get hard it is not a sign of age, but of disease, and the blood pressure goes up. 120 (systolic This is read: "120 over 85." If your blood 85 diastolic) pressure runs up to 180, that is as high as it should ever run to be on the safe side. 180 to 190 is not safe. Over 190 to 200 you are a risk; something is going to happen. If it is running 200 or over, you are an accident going someplace to happen! However, some people normally have higher blood pressure than others.

The difference between the systolic count and the diastolic count is the amount of energy that is being used by the heart in the circulation of blood in the body. The normal difference between the systolic and the diastolic reading should run between 30 and 45 points. For a person getting on in years, a difference of 45 points is not too excessive. If the heart has to use a large amount of extra energy, due to some condition in the body, this difference will run to a higher count. As an example, where a condition of hardening of the arteries exists, the heart works harder to force the blood through the arteries, and the difference between the two counts may run as high as 90 in some cases. If the count runs this high, the person is wearing out his heart very fast.

WARNING

Do not use the slanting board in cases of uterine hemorrhages, high blood pressure, or cancerous tissue. In any illness, use the slanting board only under your doctor's advice.

LOW BLOOD PRESSURE

The person with low blood pressure does not have to worry about having a stroke, but he does have to worry about having enough energy to do his job. Low blood pressure is extremely enervating. A diet high in proteins will help build up a higher blood pressure for the person suffering from this condition.

The use of the slanting board is very good in cases of low blood pressure as the blood is pulled up to the heart and head area by the position on the board. The exercises, which we will describe later on in this article, will further stimulate the circulation of the blood.

BRAIN ANEMIA

Brain anemia may be caused from overwork, and the resulting fatigue. We know that we can build two new brain cells a second, but if we are tearing down the brain cells at the rate of three a second, then we are helping to develop brain anemia. A dropped colon may also be the cause of brain anemia, as this does not allow the proper amount of calcium to be circulated through the body. Muscle tone is then not all that it should be, and the blood is not forced uphill into the brain area. The result is that every organ in the body suffers.

Every gland and organ in the body can be exhausted through lack of vital energy from the brain. There must first be blood in the brain before the fingers can go into action and play the piano. Fifteen minutes on the slanting board not only places the organs back in their proper positions, but forces the blood back into the head area, thereby regenerating the automatic brain centers; the respiratory, circulatory and gastro-intestinal centers.

Animals almost always sleep in a prone position with their head lower than the rest of their body. The eagle flies with his head below his body and his strength is tremendous. He can detect food eight to ten miles away as his senses are extremely keen and are kept that way by having the proper amount of blood in his head. If you hold a dog up for four hours, by his front legs, he will die, for his heart and arteries cannot pump enough blood into his brain to keep him alive. If you hold a rabbit up by the ears for three quarters of an hour he will die. It is necessary to have the proper amount of blood in the brain area.

Our bodies are so constructed that they normally work with this law of gravity. An example of this is the intestinal tract and the digestive system. Food follows this downward pull of gravity through the entire intestinal tract. In the ascending colon, the appendix is placed to act as an irritant, to act as an oil can, to keep the toxic material moving uphill. At the beginning of the colon, the food material is in a very liquid condition, making it easier to carry along with the peristaltic motion. In the descending colon, it uses the law of gravity to carry this toxic material downhill. Our body works with the law of gravity.

In New York City only two people were found to have sufficient calcium, out of some 4,000 cases tested. A shortage of calcium produces a lack of tone in the tissues. When we lack tone in the transverse colon, a prolapsus can develop. Having a diet rich in calcium and other minerals is a necessity in improving prolapsus.

In order to demonstrate the good that can be derived from the use of the slanting board in illness, I am going to relate a personal experience. I was very ill and one night I had a vision that opened great vistas of healing for me. I had heard the saying many times that, "The brain is the garden of the body and you can build a garden of roses or a garden of weeds from the brain." The vision, which I had the night before the crisis in my illness, is as follows:

I remember seeing myself walking along with someone in a garden. There was a large trellis above me with flowers hanging down. In the middle of the trellis was a fountain throwing water up to these flowers.

As we walked along, we came to a hose which was feeding the water into this fountain. As we approached this hose, the person alongside of me stepped on the hose, sending the water over the edge of the fountain, and the flowers withered away. I compared this situation with the blood in my head which would also wither if I did not get proper nourishment and blood to the brain. I realized that the brain was the "garden" of my body. You cannot walk, taste, or do anything physically, mentally or spiritually without the brain.

Immediately upon seeing this condition happening, I thought, "What should one do in a case like this?" The person should either get off the hose or take the fountain and place it on top of the roses, letting the water drain down on them. I recognized that if my brain needed more blood, there was one way of getting it there, and that was by putting the brain below the rest of the body, enabling the blood to flow properly.

This principle applies, first, by feeding the fatigue center which is in the topmost part of the brain. Secondly, if there is a protrusion, a prolapsed condition, this prolapsus is automatically brought back into position by the pull of gravity on the slant board. I found relief for the first time in months.

In using this board and lying in the upside-down position, I found in a period of three months I overcame my difficulties. My intestinal tract had changed entirely. Patients who use the board change their bowel activity to such an extent that those formerly having only one movement every day or two now have two or three movements daily.

What happened to me has also happened to many others through the use of this board. I am convinced of its value and necessity in a good health plan. Whenever a person becomes sick, he is tired — enervated. Anyone who is sick has lost the calcium which gives the body tone and energy, and when this tone is lost, a prolapsus can set in; that is, the transverse colon, which goes across the body, completely collapses and drops.

I have never found anyone with a perfect transverse colon. Everyone who is sick has a prolapsus. The moment a prolapsus sets in, the law of gravity causes pressure on all the organs below. The doctors have yet to know the distress and trouble that is produced in the body with the mechanical pressure of one organ bearing down on the one below through force of gravity. The more tired or ill you are, the more calcium you lack and the greater the effect gravity has on your body; the greater the mechanical pressure.

The transverse colon, which is the only soft tissue organ going from right to left across the entire body, is the first organ to feel the pull of gravity. This soft organ prolapses. When this begins to fall, the stomach falls also, causing a fishhook stomach. When prolapsus develops, we have pressure on all the organs below; the bladder, the rectum, the prostate gland, the ovaries and the kidneys. From this extra pressure, hernia and ruptures develop. Stagnant conditions of the bowel develop when the waste material is not moved along as it should be. Bowel pockets develop, gas forms, heart pressure develops, and the breathing gets out of time because of the improper diaphragm pressure and abnormal position. Curvature of the spine develops when a pot belly begins to form. The reason for this being that the potbelly comes forward and in order to hold that abnormal thing there, a curvature in the spine has to develop. When curvature of the spine develops, then there are other compensating curvatures in the upper part of the body, pulling the head back, causing the Adam's to apply to appear and creating pressure on the thyroid gland.

Consistent use of the slanting board, every day, forces these prolapsed organs back into their proper positions and eliminates the various disorders that have been caused by the prolapsus. For this one condition, the slanting board is absolutely invaluable!

BLADDER-PROSTATE

Many people, after the age of forty-five, complain about bladder disturbances. This is nothing more than a lack of energy to hold the organs in their place against the law of gravity. These people are disturbed from two to ten times a night: there is generally some condition causing irritation on the bladder. The prostate troubles are caused from prolapsus in the abdominal tract. Ninety per cent of prostate troubles are caused from prolapsus and mechanical pressure symptoms more than any disease or chemical distress.

TUMORS-UTERUS

This law of gravity pulls against the organs in women and cause distress in the form of menstrual troubles and disorders in change of life due to pressure on the ovaries and tubes. This in turn causes pressure on the uterus, forcing a malposition of the uterus, which is incapable of throwing off toxic material that has settled there. In this way a certain amount of toxic material is retained within the body, producing re-absorption of toxins.

Most fibroid tumors are caused from pressure against the uterus, which does not allow the toxic material to be eliminated from this organ. The increase in the number of fibroid tumors today is phenomenal. Many of the troubles can come from douches, but usually they come from lack of proper blood supply due to pressure from the organs above. Women who have a uterus that is tipped backward, should lie on the board face down so that the uterus is forced back into normal position.

ADHESIONS

Over a period of years, when there is a dropped transverse colon condition, these tissues begin to rub against each other and adhesions form. Adhesions do not only come from an operation; they can come from an acid condition and misplaced organs. Keep the organs active and normal.

STIFF NECK

I do not believe in using a pillow. I think it is responsible for many of our troubles today. A pillow can cause thyroid and other disturbances. It cuts off much nerve and blood supply to the brain and can cause rheumatism and neuritis. We have to teach our children to sleep on a pillow as it is not a natural inclination. After you have grown to a certain age, using a pillow, it will probably take a year to give it up entirely. Sleeping on a pillow over a period of time is conducive to producing a stiff neck. If you will try lying on a flat surface and relax, with the head completely to the side, it will keep your neck limber. Remember what the bible says: "Woe unto you who have a stiff neck."

A stiff neck keeps circulation from the brain. A relaxed, peaceful person, who has a limber neck, can look from side to side, but a greedy or jealous person does not have enough relaxation in his neck. A person with fear, money troubles or love problems, has a stiff neck. When I go over the muscles of your neck, I can tell you whether your husband, wife or mother-in-law is bothering you, or if you have financial troubles.

Nineteen million dollars were spent on laxatives last year. A great deal of this laxative buying could be stopped through the use of the board and through developing the tone of the intestinal tract. Elimination is more important than eating. When we establish normal elimination habits and continue the practice, bowel pockets get smaller and smaller. Every time we resist nature, bowel pockets get larger and the system harbors toxic poisons.

CIRCULATION IN THE LEGS

Circulation in the legs will not be good unless there is proper tone in the heart to force the blood along. We will not have proper circulation unless there is tone in the arteries, and unless we have a nerve supply originally coming from the brain to stimulate the arteries and the heart to activity. The stronger the nerve force is to those organs, the better the circulation will be. The more tired you become, the slower your circulation is.

People who bruise easily and turn blue on the slightest touch have very tired bodies. Toxic material settles there and cannot be moved along fast enough. Varicose veins are a sign of toxins which cannot be moved uphill and back again through the extremities of the body. The venous blood has very difficult time working uphill and against the pressure of the blood, when the legs are crossed. If legs were up in the air most of the time, there would be no pressure of the blood in going uphill. Most of the poor circulation is due to nerve depletion. If you have the nerve force in the brain, you will have proper circulation.

BEAUTY HINTS

"RAISE YOUR FACE FOR BEAUTY AND YOUR ORGANS FOR HEALTH." This is the saying of a famous beauty consultant and it is a world of information in a nutshell.

Leading beauty consultants all highly recommend the use of the slanting board for beauty. Beauty facials are given while the person receiving the treatment is lying on a slanting board. This causes the blood to rush to the face and neck and this extra blood, combined with the effects of the massage, makes the facial more beneficial. The position of the body on the slanting board is called "the beauty position" in these salons.

This position on the slanting board, which forces the blood into the head and neck areas, also helps to eliminate wrinkles, ear and eye conditions.

Eye exercises practiced while lying on the board are most effective. They make the eyes sparkle and are a definite part of the beauty program.

I am now going to list for you a group of exercises that you can perform on the slanting board. If you will pick out some of these exercises and use them regularly, you will see a definite improvement in your body.

BEAUTY EXERCISES

1. Blow all the air out of your lungs until you feel like a flat tire. Then, without breathing in, draw your chest up as close as you can to your chin, tensing your abdominal muscles at the same time. This exercise creates a partial vacuum in your lungs, lifts the upper part of your chest and enables suction to raise your abdominal organs into place. Notice how much smaller and flatter your stomach now looks.

Do this exercise ten times. It slims the waist, gets rid of that spare tire and gives you a streamlined front elevation.

2. Raise your right leg without bending your knee and grasp your right foot in both hands. Slowly pull your hands down foot, ankle and calf to thing, pushing up with your foot and pulling down with your hands as hard as you can.

Do this exercise five times on each leg. It not only has the same effect as Exercise One in tensing and strengthening your abdominal muscles, but also does wonders in slenderizing ankles and legs.

3. Spread your arms straight out from your shoulders, palms down. Bend your knees and bring them down to your chest. Then, still keeping your back flat on the board, knees and feet tight together, start doing figure eights as follows: Twist sideways from the waist and push your knees down to the right — a good stretch here — around and back to the knees-on-chest position, having made as big a circle as possible repeat to the left.

Do this exercise ten times. It not only restores girlish contours around the equator but is also good for constipation. After completing these exercises, rest for the balance of ten minutes — or more if you can spare the time.

GENERAL HEALTH EXERCISES

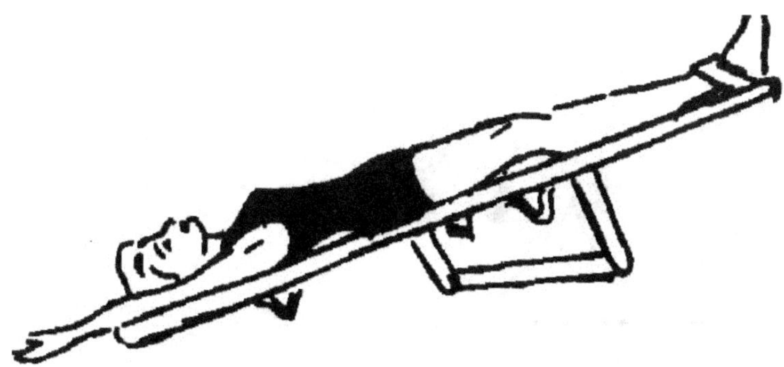

1. Stretch the arms straight above the head and stretch the spine. This allows for better circulation in the cartilages of the spine and lower organs where the blood supply may have been minimized because of pressure from the above organs.

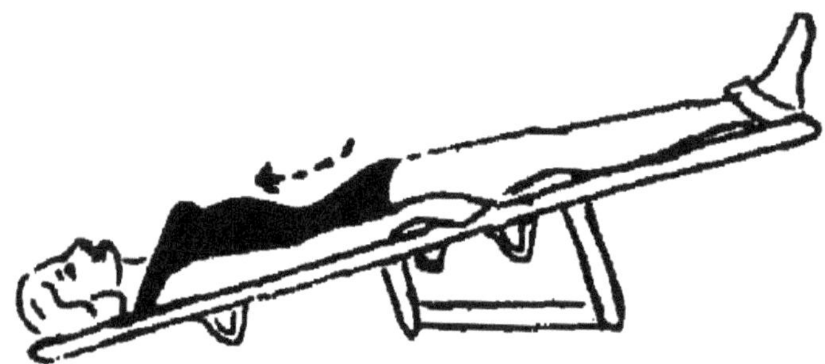

2. Pull the stomach up towards the shoulders. Pull it back and forth 10 to 15 times. Gravitation helps to keep the organs in the proper position because as you pull the intestinal organs up to the head you not only have your own force to bring them back to the proper position, but you are also using the force of gravity to help you. Do not push the stomach out.

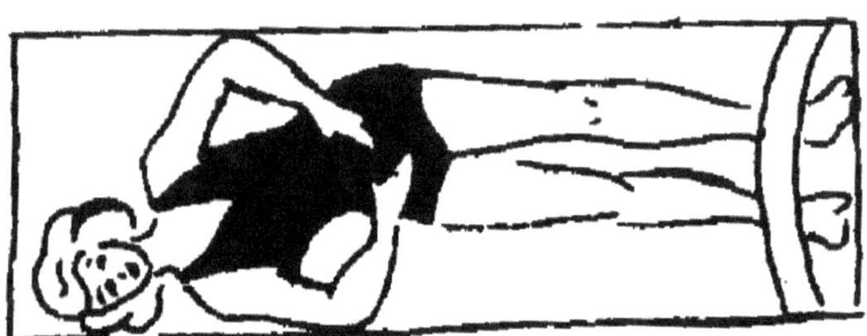

3. Pat the stomach. In patting the stomach with a fair degree of pressure or hardness you develop better circulation and bring a hyperemic condition to the abdomen. Stretch to the left side and pat on the right side. Patting the right side, when it is stretched, helps break down pockets in the intestinal tract. Do same to the left side.

This exercise will help to absorb the fat tissues in the abdomen; will develop tone in the abdominal muscles and get rid of flabbiness. Flabby muscles fall very quickly and help to produce abnormal pressure on arteries and nerves leading to the legs.

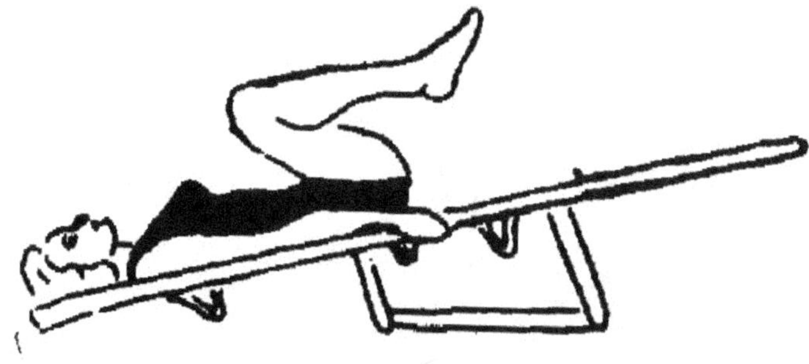

4. Remove feet from straps, flex the knees and relax. You will find a greater blood pressure in the head. In this position, the brain will get all the blood it needs for we are using gravity now to bring the blood back to the brain cells.

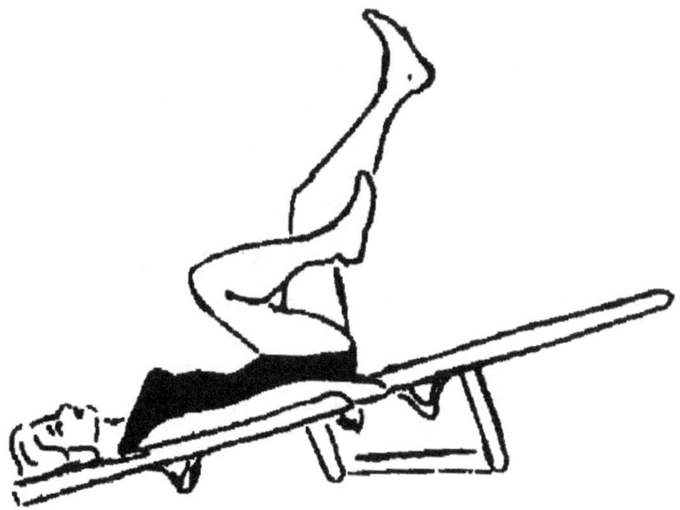

5. The bicycle exercise is a good thing for exercising

abdominal organs. Push the thighs of the legs against the abdominal organs with force to get the greatest effect. Doing the bicycle while on the floor makes you work under tension, but by doing this exercise on the slanting board you get the greatest amount of good from the gravitational pull.

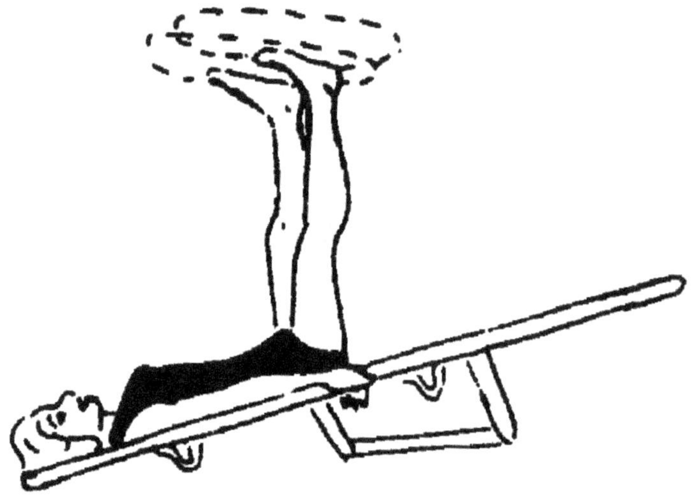

6. Lift the legs straight above the body and rotate the legs in big circles. This stretches the muscle structure of the pelvic area to allow for better circulation. It also stretches the muscles in and around the prostate gland allowing greater freedom there. This releases the pressure on the bladder and develops muscles in the lower abdomen that have not been used for a long time.

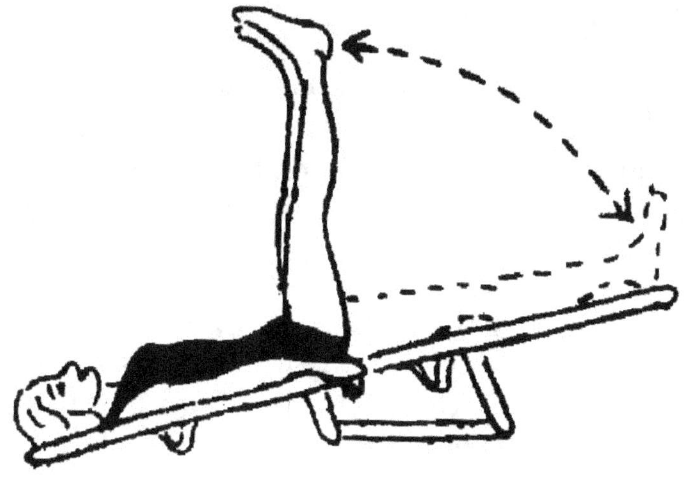

7. Bring legs straight up to vertical position and lower them to the board slowly. Repeat three or four times.

Young people, or those who desire to build up muscular strength may do these exercises with gusto, but those who are not too well or strong should use good judgment in the way they exercise, so that they do not overdo.

THE BASIC AND REST POSITION

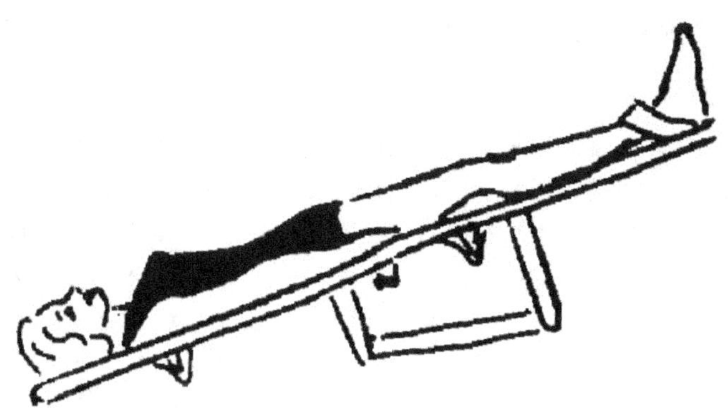

AFTER WE EXERCISE WE MUST REST

These exercises should not take more than five minutes actual time. We should lie on the board and rest in a perfectly relaxed position for at least 10 or 15 minutes. We should also rest on the board in the afternoon or before the evening meal.

You must also do these exercises just before going to bed. Doing these exercises when you are tired is most beneficial. That is the time when you can rejuvenate the fatigue centers of the brain and lift the tired soft tissue organs back into place more easily. When you have the least amount of resistance, gravity working for you can do the greatest amount of good.

The benefits of placing the head below the feet has been proven in many cases. It stands to reason that when we continue to walk around when we are dead tired, gravity can have its most disastrous results. It is the custom in the Norwegian Army to have the troops stop marching and lie down with their feet resting high on their knapsacks so that they will be able to continue the long hikes required in their training. It has been found that they recuperate faster this way and are able to walk longer distances.

These slanting board exercises, when done for a period of fifteen minutes, are equal to a good hour's rest or sleep. If a person uses the slanting board for a few minutes in the middle of the day he will have renewed energy with which to carry on his work. Regular use of the slanting board is one of the greatest "old-age preventatives" that I know of.

Real, lasting health will never be found in pill boxes or medicine bottles. There is one method, and only one, by which health can be gained and kept. That is, by assisting nature to work in her own way to cleanse and stimulate each nerve and muscle, and thus enable her marvelous recreating and rejuvenating forces to carry new life to them. Through- out life we build new tissues, new skin, nails and hair. So it is not too late — it is never too late. The human organism has powers undreamed of by most of us. Give them a chance; have faith and you will be amazed at the regeneration they can bring about in you.

"Age is quality of mind:

If you have left your dreams behind

If hope is cold,

If you no longer look ahead,

If your ambition-fires are dead,

Then you are old.

But if from life you take the best,

And if in life you keep the jest,

If love you hold,

No matter how the years go by,

No matter how the birthdays fly,

You are not old."

BEAUTY

Begin to take on beauty consciousness. See this within yourself. People are looking to you for that beauty within you. They should know you for that beauty. You should know yourself for the beauty which is possible within you. The many stages through which we go in our growth are the times when we branch out, add a few more leaves and be- come a better climber than ever before. All we need is the awareness that it is possible to have this beauty-consciousness within us; all we need is time to develop it.

The beauty was always there. It just takes a recognition within, a knowing that we can also become part of our outer expression. You walk differently, if you know that you are beautiful. Your very countenance will be different, if there is beauty within. The hardened lines of your face will soften. You will be lovelier in your greeting and will bring out the beauty of other people in their greeting. Most people are lovers of beauty. That which is expressed from the heart of beauty can be worn on anyone's face. This beauty you can wear may change the life of the people you meet to one of more beauty for them. The color of your temperament is held in this beauty within. The tension you bring back to yourself from others is produced from that which started within you. When you are expressing beauty, you not only help your neighbor, but you now express the better life yourself. Your whole body will be less tense, less confused and less chaotic.

We have to have an uplifting philosophy to keep the muscles of the face and the body in good condition. Every- thing good is felt in the very muscles of the body; every wonderful hope, aspiration, ideal is found in the sight of the eye. Likewise, every depression, disappointment, antagonism or resentment is found not only in the eye, but also in the mouth, the cheeks, the forehead. They help to make wrinkles; they are the tell-tale signs that show what kind of thinking we are indulging in. Many people claim to be happy, but they have never notified their face. Most of us come from a very poor "attitude" in life into this new way of living and now we know better. However, there are still some physical things left over that we have to overcome in our new way of life, and we have to use physical things, such as exercise, food, sunshine and air to help us attain beauty and radiant health.

Beauty comes from a healthy body. There are many things to consider in order to build this beauty. I think that iron is the most important, as far as a chemical or a mineral element is concerned. Iron gives us rich, red blood and we find, too, that the element that goes along with it is called oxygen. Iron and oxygen give us the color in our skin, and without the proper amount of this iron and oxygen in the body, we get a pasty-looking skin instead of a healthy one.

One of the finest cocktails I know for building that blush we want in our cheeks is one rich in iron made with black cherry juice and egg yolk. Any of the green tops of vegetables also give us a lot of iron. Our foods must contain the natural God given mineral elements or else our bodies will suffer and become diseased, no matter how much good natural protein and starch we may have. We must have the mineral foods as a balance to metabolize the starches, proteins and fats.

Muscle tone is built from within. When there is a lack of muscle tone, the jowls will drop, the cheek muscles will begin to droop, and eventually there will be two or three chins. This condition is the result of lack of exercise, good air, and faulty or improper body metabolism.

The natural bloom that should be on the cheeks that little bloom of youth that is found on a child's face and which we would all like to carry with us throughout life, cannot be there if we work too hard, exhaust our nervous systems, worry and have an unbalanced diet. We should also get the proper amount of sleep, so that our bodies can repair and rebuild themselves.

Sleep is the greatest medicine of all. Rest really cures and beautifies. Just as plants, flowers, trees grow at night, so does our beauty. Therefore, proper rest is most essential, and can be had best, if we use the slant board before retiring, so that the body is put in its best natural alignment. And stay in bed one day a week, or as often as is possible, and save your heart 2,000 beats. Be kind to your body and your body will be kind to you.

To have beauty to its fullest extent, we must also depend on the right kind of exercise. To put good food into the body and allow it to stagnate through a lack of exercise, will not help us to attain the bloom of youth that we want to have, particularly as we get older. The slanting board exercises help to give us more color in our face and bring our complexion back to normal quicker than anything else. The slanting board brings more blood to the head, face, hair and eyes. It gives the hair both luster and sheen and gives a gleam to the eye, as every tissue in the head gets the proper supply of blood. So we become more alive when 'we use the slanting board. We all need to have well-nourished tissues for vibrant health.

The tissues in the upper part or head area begin to deteriorate first, when our body becomes tired and depleted. When we have a tired body, gravity keeps us from forcing the blood supply up into the head and so our beauty begins to leave us. First, our color begins to leave our face; then the eyes begin to look dull, and soon we find that our teeth begin to crumble and get bad; they begin to discolor and crake with white spots in them, showing that we lack certain chemical elements in the body. So, if you want to recover your waning or disappearing beauty, the slanting board exercises are the finest things to help the body normalize the circulation.

Try to take daily air baths. Of course you may wear a very light and loose garment, but nothing is more invigorating than to have a current of air strike the bare skin. Get a ventilator or a window that admits air without creating a draft. Air baths invigorate the skin and improve the circulation. Also take the skin brushing bath. This is the cleanest bath I know. It helps the nerves and the elimination of catarrh, nerve acids and uremic acids from the circulation and system. The skin is an organ of elimination. A natural bristle brush (not nylon) should be used at least once a day, preferably in the morning — to give a four to five minute flesh massage. This may be repeated before going to bed.

Sun baths are beneficial and should be taken during the seasons which make them possible. Most people are lacking in calcium and sun baths will "fix" the calcium in the organs and various parts of the body where it is needed. The sun carries the power and energy to distribute calcium into every tissue of the body, helping to give it tone. Do not sunbathe in the extreme heat of the day and start with only ten minutes, gradually increasing until you can comfortably stay for one hour.

A beautiful skin must be an active skin. All the muscles underlying the skin must become firm. They will become firm. They will become so through exercises and through feeding them proper material from the blood. Watch your diet. Make good blood, which in turn will make better skin. New skin is underneath ready to take the place of the old as soon as it drops off but remember that the skin underneath can be no better than the blood from which it is made. There is no skin condition that cannot be changed and made better by following a natural living regime.

One of the best things for the skin is Oat Straw Tea, which contains silicon.

HERE IS THE RECIPE:

Take 1/2 cup of oat straw to 2-1/2 cups of water. Boil 7 to 10 minutes (or follow instructions on package) Silicon is not lost by boiling. Strain and drink this amount daily. Add lemon to flavor, honey to sweeten.

A WONDERFUL SKIN TONIC

One green pepper (rich in Vitamin C) finely chopped, 1/2 cup Oat Straw Tea to 1 quart of water. Simmer for 40 minutes — strain off. Drink one cup — 2 or 3 times daily.

FOR COMPLEXION GLOW

1/3 cup Strawberry Juice, 1/3 cup Rhubarb Juice, I Slice of Fresh Pineapple, Dash of Honey. Blend till smooth.

FOR SKIN BRACER

1 Tbsp. Apple Concentrate

1/2 Cup Water

1/2 Cup Cucumber Juice

TRY A HONEY PACK

For the face. Place a little honey in a small dish. Put some honey on the fingers and then pat the face and neck, wherever any wrinkles appear. Let the honey pull on the skin as you pull away from it. The pulling away will exercise the skin and give the tissues underneath the tone to build and smooth the skin. The honey also softens and cleanses the skin. Do these five minutes daily. Wash the honey off with warm water and finish with cold water.

Try to put your body in order and then you will have a good skin. Also give your face a chance to breathe and the nighttime is the best opportunity you have to give your skin a rest and time to breathe.

Sometimes an oldish appearance of the face can come about prematurely, if a person does not drink enough water every day. The fullness and the roundness of the face is usually due to the amount of fluids that it contains. When the fluids are lacking the face may appear lean and haggard and the skin folded and shriveled. The amount of water that the average person should consume in twenty-four hours is a minimum of three pints (or about six glasses.)

And along with the other exercises, don't forget that the best exercise for the face is to smile, smile, smile.

Always try to eat as natural food as possible and make a habit of applying the following general diet regimen to your everyday living. This is a healthy way to live and health is the basis of real beauty. You do not have to think of vitamins, mineral elements or calories, if you have two different fruits every day, at least 4 to 6 vegetables, with one protein, one starch and either a fruit or vegetable juice between meals. Eat at least two green leafy vegetables. Consider this procedure to be a dietetic law.

Always keep cheerful when eating, as cheerfulness stimulates the gastric secretions. A good thing to remember is: "First eat what your body needs, then eat what you like if you must."

You should learn what supplementary foods need to be added to your diet to keep you in perfect health. For instance, there is whey, which is a great dissolver and one of the highest sodium foods we can use. It is good to use in all digestive disturbances. Sodium is the chemical element that keeps joints limber, active, pliable — it is what we call the "youth" element. Use whey every day. Get the powder and put it in your drinks, your soups or sprinkle on salads. Celery tablets and okra tablets are also high in sodium.

Take dulse tablets for iodine necessary to the thyroid gland, which controls the metabolism and the weight in the body. Have foods that are rich in potassium. Make drinks from the green tops of vegetables, as this is good to tone the tissues. Also have wheat germ oil, lecithin and gelatin and try to have 2 tablespoons of sunflower seed meal four times a day in a drink, in soup or sprinkled on a salad.

Learn the value of Herbal Teas. Mint teas are good as aids in digestion; Oat straw tea carries the property of feeding silicon to the body for the care of veins in the legs, feet or hands and it gets rid of dry skin. Bran tea is very high in silicon and will help people who want to get the gloss back into their hair; it also helps a poor skin condition.

Taking flaxseed tea or a tablespoonful of flaxseed meal daily will help the skin tone and also improve the health of the hair tremendously. It seems to prevent grey hair and also gives the hair a desirable sheen. Don't forget that hair needs sunshine and fresh air and that it must be fed 'from the inside at mealtime. Blood streams carry nourishment to the hair so supply your blood stream with the necessary foods or nutrition. Exercise the scalp by rubbing it at least ten minutes each day. Shampoo one week to ten days apart.

FOR HAIR SHEEN

1 tsp. Cherry Concentrate

1 Cup Oat Straw Tea

Sip Slowly

HAIR BEAUTIFYING COCKTAIL

2/3 Cup Oat Straw Tea

1 /3 Celery, or prune, or fig juice

1 /4 tsp. Powdered Nova Scotia Dulse to each cup

AFTER SHAMPOO

2 eggs with 1/2 tsp. sea salt mixed together. Rub well into scalp, then rinse off with almost cool water.

Alfalfa or Parsley tablets are good to take for restoring color to grey hair.

COFFEE BREAK

When you have a "coffee break" make it a "broth break" and have a pause that profits.

1 tsp. Vegetable Seasoning (broth powder)

1 tsp. Whey Powder

1/2 tsp. Dulse Powder

In one cup of hot water

As this beauty business goes to the mental side of life also, I feel that all the work you do on the outside of the body is of no avail until you think Beautiful thoughts within. When you are beautiful within, it is going to start working itself out on the surface.

It is very important to realize that beauty is a Godly quality and that the person who has a beautiful countenance must have a beautiful soul. If people could allow the beauty from within to come out, they would have fewer wrinkles, the hard marks on the face would begin to leave and they would find that while beauty can be patched up, it also can be developed.

Beautiful thoughts within and a perfectly working physical and mental body is more important in building vibrant Beauty than anything you can do to the outside of the body. We should remember that the most perfectly groomed person with a frown on his countenance does not give an impression of vibrant good health, which after all is the most beautiful thing we can express physically. "Beauty is as Beauty does," and to me, the most commonplace person with good manners and good health is truly a blessing to all who behold such a person. We can all be beautiful in our own way!

For that glow of health, use the beautifying, tried and tested recipes, along with suggested arrangements, originated at Hidden Valley Health Center, appearing on the following pages.

DRINK SUGGESTIONS NO. 1

MILKY WHEY

2 Tbsp Whey Powder

1 Glass Milk (raw)

Few drops Vanilla

1 Tbsp Cashews

2 Tbsp Coconut

Blend: Sprinkle with nutmeg.

HERCULES PUNCH

1/2 C Apple Juice

1/2 C Papaya Juice

1 tsp Wheat Germ Oil

1 tsp Lecithin Granules

1 tsp Bone Meal

1 tsp Brewer's Yeast 1 tsp Skim Milk Powder

Blend in liquefier to smooth consistency.

RADIANCE COCKTAIL

1/2 C Celery Juice

1/2 C Orange Juice

1 tsp Raw Almond Butter

Whipped in.

NERVE-VERVE

1 C Prune Juice

6 Radishes

2 tsp Rice Polishing

JADE-ADE

1/4 C Cucumber Juice

1/4 C Watercress Juice

1/4 C Celery Juice

1/4 C Tomato Juice

1/4 C Parsley Juice

MOC-CHOC-MILK

2 Tbsp Carob

1/4 C Water

(Cream. Heat in a double boiler until thick, stirring occasionally.)

2 C Milk

2 Tbsp Honey

1/2 tsp Pure Vanilla

Add and re-heat until hot enough for a drink. A dash of whipped cream on top.)

DRINK SUGGESTIONS NO. 2

NERVE TONER

Pineapple Juice

1 Egg Yolk

1 tsp Rice Polishing

APPLE ZIP

I Glass Apple Juice

1 Egg Yolk

1/4 tsp Powdered Dulse

YOUTH BLOOM

1/3 C Beet Juice

1/3 C Spinach Juice

2 Tbsp Blackberries

Liquefy

YOGURT FLIP

1 C Yogurt

Juice of 1/2 Lemon

1 tsp Chlorophyll

Little Dulse Powder

Little Honey

Few drops of Vanilla

TROPICAL MINT TEA

1/2 C Orange Juice

1/2 C Lemon Juice

1/4 C Papaya Juice

2 C Mint Tea

1 Beaten Egg White

Serve in 3 tall glasses with cherries on sticks

HORS D'OEUVRE NOVELTIES

Celery stuffed with Nut Butter

Celery stuffed with Cheese

Cheese Balls

Sunflower Seeds

Melon Seeds

Raw, unsalted Nuts

Black Olives

Tender young cabbage leaves filled with: Nut butters, Cheese, Cottage Cheese, Tofu or Egg. Garnish with pimento or pepper slices.

GREEN PEPPER STRIPS

Spread with cream cheese and dipped in Chlorophyll tinted Coconut.

1 C. Finely Ground Almonds, 2 tsp. Egg White, Honey to blend. Mix well. Roll into balls in coconut.

1 Slice Rye Bread, Layer of Avocado (sprinkle with lemon juice), Spread with cottage cheese. Sprinkle with vegetable seasoning, Stand on an upright square of alfalfa sprouts, Garnish with favorite dressing.

Baby Green and Yellow Summer Squash sliced thinly. Sandwich in odd pairs with squares of sharp cheese between. Secure with toothpicks.

LIGHT FANTASTICKS

Arrange attractively an assortment of: Carrot Sticks, Celery Sticks, Cucumber Sticks, Green and Red Pepper Sticks, Zucchini Sticks, Sliced Jerusalem Artichokes, Sliced Radishes Black Olives — And use with your favorite spread — placed in a handy dish.

SOUPS

MINT-GREEN COOL SOUP

1 C Unsweetened Pineapple Juice

1 C Strong Mint Tea

2 tsp Gelatin

1/4 C Peppermint Leaves

1 Tbsp Apple Concentrate

1 Very Ripe Banana

Blend till very fine and smooth.

BROTH DELICIOSO

1 C Sesame Milk — Heat without boiling.

2 tsp Vegetable Seasoning — dissolve in

1 Tbsp Boiling Water

1 Tbsp Finely Chopped Parsley

Mix — Serve in hot soup bowls.

CREAMED-GREEN WARM-UP

1/2 C Fresh or Frozen Uncooked Peas, or Spinach,

or Broccoli

1 C Vegetable Broth

1 Sprig Mint

1 tsp Vegetable Seasoning

1/2 tsp Raw Sugar

Few Sprigs Watercress or Parsley

Liquefy until very smooth. Heat over boiling water until serving temperature is reached.

ADD: 2 Tbsp Raw Cream — and serve.

SALADS AND A LUNCH IDEA

BEAUTY QUEEN LUNCH

1 C Pineapple Juice

1/2 C Orange Juice

1 Prune, soaked and pitted

1 /2 C Walnuts

1/4 C Sunflower Seeds

1 Small Carrot, diced

1/4 C Alfalfa Sprouts

2 Sprigs Parsley

Dash Celery Salt

1 Leaf Comfrey

1/2 Ripe Banana

1 Egg

2 Tbsp Wheat Germ

Blend all the ingredients at same time. Put in a thermos over crushed ice and take to work for a quick 'beauty' lunch. Drink slowly through a straw.

FAN SHAPED SALAD

Cut Apples (with red skins) and Pears into 1 /8ths. Alternate in groups of 3, sandwiching a soft blue cheese in between. Spread out fan-fashion. Place on a bed of crisp Romaine. Serve with a light cream dressing. Garnish with Watercress or Parsley.

LIVING GREEN SALAD

1 Cucumber — diced

1 Green Pepper — chopped fine

1 Bunch Radishes — sliced

1 Green Onion

Few Sprigs Watercress

Few Sprigs Parsley

1 Tbsp Lemon Juice

4 Tbsp Virgin Olive Oil

1 tsp Vegetable Seasoning

Shake together in a bottle

Toss salad in dressing. Serve on Romaine Leaves.

AVOCADO DELIGHT

Watercress

1/2 Avocado

Cottage Cheese

Tomato Slices

Sunflower Seeds

Fill avocado with cottage cheese. Arrange on watercress, circle with tomato slices and garnish with sunflower seeds.

"EAT-YOUR-FILL" DRESSING

1C Yogurt

1/2 C Blue Cheese, crumbled

Mix together lightly.

FOR THAT "SWEET TOOTH"

PERSIMMON DREAM

2 Very Ripe Persimmons, pureed

1 C Whipped Cream

Serve on Sundae dishes, garnishing with a half walnut.

SEA FOAM

I Tbsp Gelatin soften

1 Tbsp Cold Water

1 C Boiling Water

Add and dissolve

1/3 C Raw Sugar — stir in

1 C Pineapple Juice

1/4 C Lime Juice

1 tsp Chlorophyll

Add: (almost allow to set)

1 Egg White. Beat in very thoroughly

Chill until firm.

PRUNE WHIP

1 C Pureed Prunes

1 Tbsp Honey

Dash of Nutmeg

Little Grated Lemon Rind

1 C Yogurt

Fold gently together. Serve in Sundae dishes topped with grated nuts.

BANANA MANNA

1 C Sesame Milk

1 Banana

Few Chopped Dates

Little Papaya, if desired

Chill

APPLE TANGY

1 C Yogurt

1 Ripe, Sweet Apple

2 tsp Orange Juice

A little orange rind

2 tsp Gelatin

Honey to sweeten

Top with Nutmeg

BAKED APPLE DE LUXE

Bake an Apple in the usual way, stuffing plentifully with dates. When ready to serve, make sauce:

1 Tbsp Nut Butter

1/4 C of the Apple Juice

Beat or blend till creamy. Serve over apple.

DATE-SWEET

12 Dates, soft

3 Tbsp Sunflower Seed Meal

Honey to blend

Stuff the Dates

Use instead of candies

MOC-CHOC SAUCE

4 Sqs. Carob-Chocolate, cut up

1/2 C Raw Sugar

1/2 C Hot Milk or Cream

1 tsp Pure Vanilla

Dash of Sea Salt

Blend smooth.

STRAWBERRY COUPE

1 C Strawberries or Raspberries, pureed

1/4 C Honey

1 C Whipped Cream

Fold together lightly. Serve in Sundae dishes, topped with a shaking of coconut.

HOW TO USE THE SLANTING BOARD

For best results, exercise on the board just after rising, before meals and before retiring, and always on an empty stomach. During the exercise wear few clothes as possible and be sure there is fresh air in the room. Specifically slanting board exercises are given to strength and bring back into normal position prolapsed abdominal and pelvic organs. If a person does nothing more than lie on the Slanting Board, the force of gravity will pull the organs back into position, thus allowing normal nerve and blood supply to nourish these organs.

Exercises taken while lying in this position build muscle and tissue tone to maintain these organs in their proper position. Cases of hernia have been corrected or improved through these exercises (exceptions noted).

SLANTING BOARD exercises are also excellent for general body building. They build muscle tone and vitality. They help to normalize circulation, glandular activity and all other metabolic processes.

Most any carpenter can make one of these boards with the illustrations given here as a guide, though some put an ordinary belt around an ironing board with one end on a chair and use this "makeshift."

DIRECTIONS

There are three Slanting Board positions, namely; Reclining, Side (either left or right) and Prone. All exercises are taken in one of these positions.

GOOD FORM IS NECESSARY. In all straight arm exercises keep the elbows and fingers straight. In all straight leg exercises keep the knees straight and the toes pointed. TENSE THE MUSCLES during the movements of each exercise.

RELAXATION is just as important as the exercise itself. Relaxation allows the blood, ladened with fatigue poisons to leave the muscle and blood filled with new nourishment to take its place. Therefore rest between exercises for an instant and never become more than comfortably tired. Fifteen minutes is enough to exercise at one time.

A beginner usually executes each selected exercise from three to six times, gradually increasing the number of times as strength and endurance increases. Confine yourself to the lighter exercises (which are given in the beginning of each GROUP) until you can do them with ease. ADD new exercises from each GROUP one at a time. In this way every fiber in the muscle is gradually strengthened and strain prevented.

WARNING: Heart and high blood pressure cases should not take these exercises unless under professional supervision.

Prolapsed abdominal and pelvic organs and hernia cases should not take full sitting positions. Such exercises are so marked.

GROUP ONE

LIE ON BACK — HEAD AT LOWER END, FEET UNDER THE STRAP, ARMS ON TABLE AT SIDES.

1. Raise right arm forward and upward overhead — keeping elbows and fingers straight. Same with left arm. Alternate one at a time. Alternate continuously. Now both together. Extend right arm sideward and

upward overhead — keeping arm at level with the body. Same with left arm. Alternate one at a time. Alternate continuously. Now both together.

2. Raise head touching chin to chest. Face right and raise head (keeping face turned to the right). Same facing left.

3. Elbows on table at sides. Raise hips as high as you can — weight on back of head, elbows, shoulders, and heels.

4. Elbows on tables at sides. Raise trunk to half-sitting position. Weight on elbows and buttocks.

5. Arms overhead. Raise to a full sitting position — throwing the arms forward at the same time. Touch the toes if possible. Same exercise keeping the arms folded.

6. Try it keeping the fingers clasped behind the neck, touching opposite knee with the elbows, one at a time while sitting. Eventually try this exercise with arms remaining stretched overhead. NOTE: NOT FOR PROLAPSED CONDITIONS AND HERNIA.

GROUP TWO

FEET OUT FROM UNDER STRAP. HANDS CLASPING HAND RAILS.

1. Flex right heel, bringing heel to buttocks — foot resting on table. Same with left knee. Alternate one at a time. Alternate continuously. Now both legs together (vary this by spreading knees wide apart and closing while the knees are flexed.

2. Bring heels to buttocks and raise hips as high as possible — weight on shoulders and feet.

3. Flex right knee to chest — toe pointed. Same with the left leg. Alternate one at a time. Alternate continuously. Now both at a time.

4. Raise right leg overhead. Same with left leg. Alternate one at a time. Alternate continuously. Now both together. Raise right leg to right angle with the body. Circumduct the leg — making as large a circle as possible — first one way then the other. Same with the left leg.

5. Raise the left leg overhead. Roll the body to the right, touching toe to the floor. Same with the right leg. Alternate.

6. Above — Raise both legs to right angle with the body. Make the scissors movement. This is done by spreading the legs wide apart, then crossing them in front of the body — first one leg in front then the other.

7. Raise to a full sitting position — feet wide apart under the strap, hands on hips. Twist the trunk from side to side. While in sitting lean the trunk from side to side. Circumduct the trunk making as large a circle as possible.   NOTE   NOT   FOR   PROLAPSED CONDITIONS AND HERNIA.

8. Raise both legs to right angle with the body. Do the bicycle movement. Use the same movement used in peddling a bicycle. Raise both legs to right angle to the body. Lower both legs together as far as possible — first to the right and then to the left. Raise both legs to right angle to the body. Circumduct the legs — first one way then the other — making as large a circle as possible.

9. Rest body on shoulders, hips high off the table. Now do the bicycle and scissors movements.

10. Raise both legs up and over the head, touching toes to the floor. Increase the distance over the head gradually in order to prevent a neck injury.

GROUP THREE

LIE FACE DOWN, FEET UNDER THE STRAP AND ARMS ON TABLE AT SIDES.

1. Raise arms upward as far as possible.

2. Extend arms straight out from shoulders and left straight up. Arms overhead. Raise the arms and shoulders, arching the back.

3. Interlace the fingers behind the back. Pull hard toward your feet, straightening the arms, raising the shoulders and arching the back. (In this exercise the head should be kept on a level with the body or back.) This will help to correct round shoulders due to too much curve in the spine.

GROUP FOUR

LIE ON LEFT SIDE, LEFT FOOT UNDER THE STRAP, LEFT ARM UNDER THE HEAD, AND RIGHT ARM ON RIGHT SIDE. BODY AND LEGS STRAIGHT.

1. Flex right arm bringing right hand to the shoulder — fist closed. Position — fingers straight.

2. Flex right knee to chest — toe pointed. Now flex arm and knee together.

3. Swing the right arm forward and backward across the body as far as you can reach. Swing right leg forward and backward as far as you can reach. Alternate exercises 3 and 4 by bringing the arm forward and the leg backward at the same time and vice versa.

4. Raise right arm side upward. Raise right leg side upward. Raise the arm and leg together.

5. Place the right hand on the table in front of the chest. Press trunk up to a half-leaning position — weight on right hand and left elbow. Right hand on hip. Both feet under the strap — one ahead of the other. Raise hips as high as possible.

6. Both feet under the strap — one ahead of the other. Assume a full side-leaning position — trunk resting on left hand (arm straight), and left hip. With right hand

on hip, raise as high as you can and lower. Same exercise done while lying on the right side.

GROUP FIVE

FEET OUT FROM UNDER THE STRAP. HANDS ON HANDRAILS.

1. Flex left knee bringing heel to buttock. Same with right knee. Alternate one at a time. Alternate continuously. Now both together.

2. Raise the right leg upward. Same with left leg. Alternate one at a time. Alternate continuously. Now both together. Swing the right leg across the left leg as far as possible by rolling up on left hip — giving the spine a good twist. Same with left leg. Alternate.

FEET UNDER THE STRAP

3. Place hands on table in front of shoulders. Push up until the arms are straight and the back arched — hips on table.

4. Hands on table in front of shoulders. Do Rocking Horse exercise. Rise on hands and knees and let the body go back until the buttocks touch the heels and your head is between your arms. Lower the chest as near the table as you can. Rock back and forth. NOTE:

This exercise is especially good for retroversion's.

5. Hands in front of shoulders. Rise on hands and toes — back straight.

Someday try lowering the chest and touching your nose to the table and raise again without touching the table with the body.

"We should all look our very best. To do this takes constant application of right living habits. To give our body the proper muscle tone and to keep it in good trim you will find the slanting board your best friend."

— ROBBIE WHITE

OTHER BOOKLETS BY DR. JENSEN

1. HOW TO ENJOY BETTER HEALTH FROM NATURAL REMEDIES

2. HOW TO RELAX AND RELIEVE TENSION

3. HOW TO REVITALIZE YOUR GLANDS

4. A NEW SLANT ON HEALTH AND BEAUTY—SLANT BOARD

5. A HEALTH PATTERN TO LIVE BY

6. HOW TO BUILD A BETTER BODY FROM YOUR KITCHEN

7. HOW THE BREATH OF LIFE SUSTAINS YOU

8. PHYSICAL, MENTAL AND SPIRITUAL BALANCE

9. DEVELOPING INWARD CALM

10. THE NEED FOR A NEW ATTITUDE

11. THE HEART AND THE CIRCULATORY SYSTEM

12. THREE STEPS TO THE HIGHER LIFE (Part I)

13. THREE STEPS TO THE HIGHER LIFE (Part II)

14. THREE STEPS TO THE HIGHER LIFE (Part III)

15. HEALTH FOR OUR CHILDREN

16. SPECIAL FOODS FOR SPECIAL NEEDS

17. LETS BEGIN AT THE BEGINNING

18. YOUR LOVE LIFE

19. INTESTINAL DISORDERS & FASTING & ELIMINATIVE DIETS

20. VOLUME I — SECRETS I CAN SHARE WITH YOU

21. VOLUME II — MORE SECRETS I CAN SHARE WITH YOU

MEET THE AUTHOR

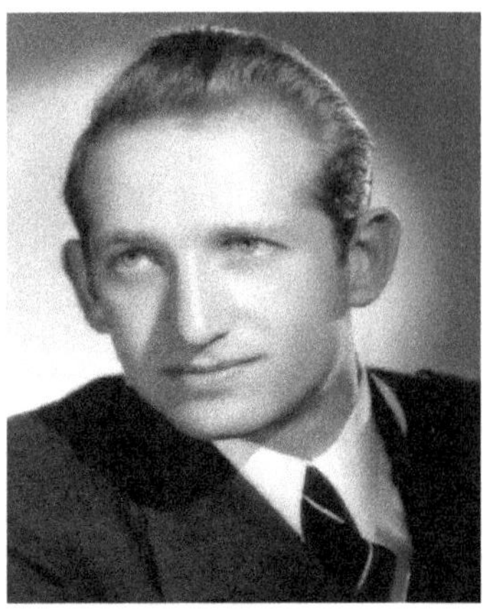

Bernard Jensen, Ph.D., D.C, N.D., Nutritionist of Los Angeles, Calif. Born in Stockton, Calif, in 1908.

Possessing a convincing philosophy that would credit much older practitioners, Bernard Jensen, D.C, Lecturer and Teacher of Right Living, acquired from the beginning of his studies the vision "that Nature does all the healing." He believes doctors can only work with natural laws. His work is sane, up-to-date, practical and teaches a balanced "how-to-live" regime.

At only 18, Dr. Jensen began studies with the West Coast Chiropractic College, Oakland, Calif. At 21 he began his practice of chiropractic in that city and has been practicing that science ever since. Widely traveled, he has been honored with post-graduate degrees from the National College in Chicago and the American School of Naturopathy, New York. He studied methods of the Battle Creek Sanitarium, of Tilden's School of Fasting in Denver. At an early age he was teaching his "How-to-live" methods to professional groups.

For 50 years. Dr. Jensen has led a most strenuous life, lecturing, radio broadcasting and directing his own health center in Escondido, California.

His current plans include Radio and TV guest appearances, a nationwide tour, and more contributions to Iridology and color, with new works planned in both areas. Dr. Jensen's The Science and Practice of Iridology has brought him international acclaim and is currently being translated into Spanish. Nine more books are in various stages of production, including his spiritual masterpiece. Arise and Shine, and color book.

ABOUT THE AUTHOR

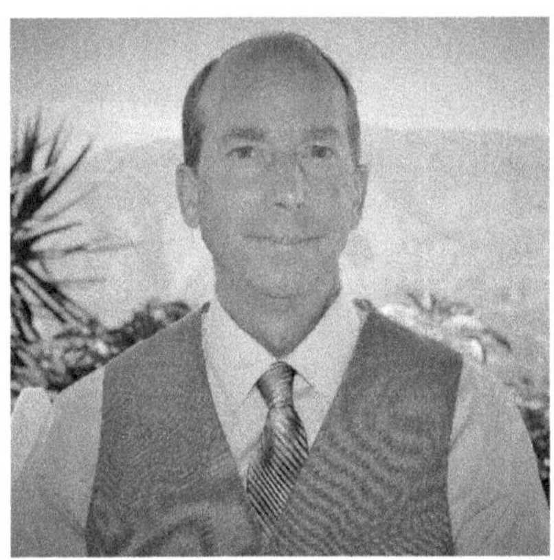

Jon Jensen, Iridologist, CMH, has been involved in holistic health for over 30 years with experience in Iridology, nutrition, and personal self-development. Jon started taking classes in Iridology and nutrition from his grandfather, the late Dr. Bernard Jensen, in 1980. Dr. Bernard Jensen is generally regarded throughout North America as the forefather of Iridology. Jon filled numerous roles over the years and participated in his grandfather's many classes and projects. Jon was involved in research for his grandfather's books, helping to pioneer a new way of iris analysis using the computer, and assisting with seminars.

Jon's mission is to educate people on the basic tenants of health and nutrition that his grandfather taught throughout his lifetime as a holistic health practitioner. Basics like the importance of a plant-based diet, regular exercise, proper sleep/rest, taking care of the bowel and more. Throughout his travels he searched for the longest living humans and wanted to know why they lived so long.

In 1995 Jon stayed by his grandfather's side after Dr. Bernard Jensen became paralyzed from the waist down from a car accident. Jon was right there every day of his grandfather's plan to walk again. With a big sign on the wall in front of Dr. Jensen's bed where he could see it every day that said, "LUCKY BOY". Every day consisted of many different healing modalities and supplements. Jon would travel to the Hidden Valley Health Ranch in the early morning and watch while Apolinar, Dr. Jensen's main ranch worker, milked the goat for Dr. Jensen's fresh morning goat milk drink. Jon would drive his grandfather and grandmother Marie to Los Angeles twice a week for chiropractic adjustments and frequency therapy, treating the whole body, mind, and spirit, and being involved in every aspect of what the doctors called a **"Miracle"—as his grandfather walked again on his own.** Jon is writing more on the entire recovery process and will publish it through Amazon.

After his grandfather's recovery, Jon shifted his attention to additional training by taking classes with some of the prominent leaders in the fields of Sclerology with Dr. Leonard Mehlmauer, Rayid (emotional iridology) with Denny Johnson, European based integrated iridology with Dr. Ellen Tart-Jensen as well as animal iridology with Dr. Mercedes Colburn.

Jon attended Kalos© classes with Dr. Valerie Seeman-Gersch learning about Transformational Healing methods.

Jon was President of the Escondido Chapter of Chamber Toastmasters and enjoys speaking to groups.

Jon has given presentations at: Holistic Health Fairs, Expo's, Herb Shops, Churches and Health Food Stores.

Jon is currently Executive Director at the "Live Pure Kids" foundation in Arizona. Jon works closely with Gavin Tucker the President/Founder, and Jackie Morales, Vice President.

The Live Pure Kids Foundation

Mission Statement: To change the world for our next generation starting from within.

Vision Statement: With the support of parents, families and the community, educating all kids through an organic plant-based mindfulness yoga lifestyle, we are giving our next generation the tools of today to be the world leaders of tomorrow.

www.livepurekids.com

Jon recently published a nutrition book called, "A Simple Guide to Healthy Living" along with the 21 Dr. Jensen Booklet series and they are available for purchase on Amazon.

For more information Jon can be found at www.jensenholistichealth.com www.bernardjensen.org